Clean Eating

Your Guide To Eating Clean
$^*2^{nd}$ Edition–Over 30 Recipes Added

Daisy Williams

I want to dedicate this book to anyone who is new to clean eating or interested in the concept of clean eating.

Speedy Publishing LLC (c) 2014
40 E. Main St., #1156
Newark, DE 19711
www.speedypublishing.co

Ordering Information:
Quantity sales; Special discounts are available on quantity purchases by corporations, associations, and others. For details, contact the "Special Sales Department" at the address above.

-- 2nd edition

Manufactured in the United States of America

Table of Contents

PUBLISHER'S NOTES

Disclaimer

This publication is intended to provide helpful and informative material. It is not intended to diagnose, treat, cure, or prevent any health problem or condition, nor is intended to replace the advice of a physician. No action should be taken solely on the contents of this book. Always consult your physician or qualified health-care professional on any matters regarding your health and before adopting any suggestions in this book or drawing inferences from it.

The author and publisher specifically disclaim all responsibility for any liability, loss or risk, personal or otherwise, which is incurred as a consequence, directly or indirectly, from the use or application of any contents of this book.

Any and all product names referenced within this book are the trademarks of their respective owners. None of these owners have sponsored, authorized, endorsed, or approved this book.

Always read all information provided by the manufacturers' product labels before using their products. The author and publisher are not responsible for claims made by manufacturers.

Print Edition 2014

CHAPTER 1: WHAT IS CLEAN EATING?

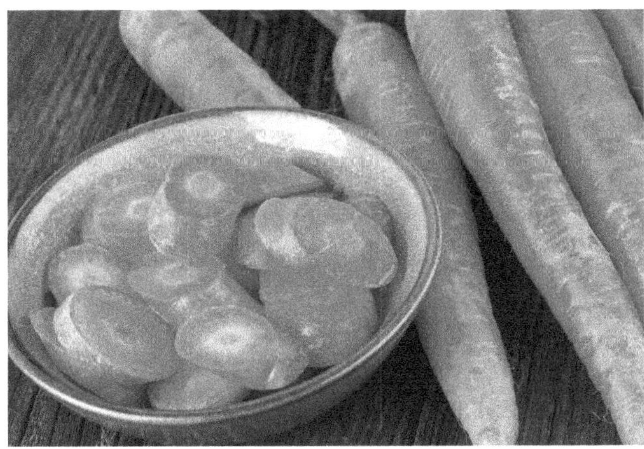

There is no way you can become healthy and without eating healthy. No matter how often or how long you exercise, you will not get anywhere without clean eating.

Your body confirms it. If you choose to eat healthy, fresh, whole foods, you will radiate health and energy.

People who simply want to detox and remove chemicals from their bodies and their diets should eat clean. The focus is not on reducing body weight, but on overall health. Processed food of all kinds should be avoided.

The focus here is on eating foods directly from nature, especially leafy greens. Avoid the foods that have been altered by humans (food manufacturers) in any form.

Eat whole meats that come directly from a butcher. Prepackaged meats can come with additives that may be harmful to the body. If at all possible, purchase whole meat and grind it yourself. (Upon request, a good butcher can grind meat you have purchased.)

Have your grains and enjoy them. Eat the ones that are whole. Replace white rice with brown rice, and eat whole grains like whole wheat.

Ensure that you read the labels of every food you purchase. If you see refined white flour in the list, it is not a clean food.

Eat foods with fewer ingredients. Ensure that you recognize all of the ingredients individually. If there is a spice listed, contact the company to verify that their listing refers to natural spices and herbs. If not, stay away. If you cannot pronounce an ingredient, it is most likely a chemical and it should be avoided. (Natural foods taste so much better anyway!

Eat 5 or 6 small meals every day. At first, this might seem like too much, but bear in mind that the portions you are eating will be smaller. If you're struggling, get your three meals as well as snacks ready for the day and divide your dinner and lunch in half. You'll get six smaller meals.

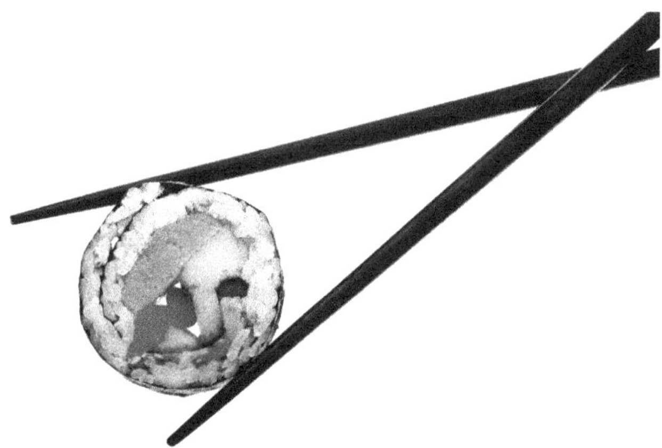

You might find clean eating a little overwhelming when you first start, particularly if you are making big changes. It is suggested that you start with baby steps. Make small changes to make the process easier. Don't beat yourself up if you make mistakes.

General Information to Help You Get Started

People who are accustomed to eating processed foods will find it difficult at first to deal with the natural flavors. People who primarily eat processed food usually say they do not like vegetables or healthy choices. However, tastes do change with time. After eating clean food for just a few weeks, many people who allow themselves a “cheat” day find processed food dull and disappointing.

CHAPTER 2: HOW TO REMOVE CHEMICALS AND HORMONES FROM YOUR DIET

When you are trying to take steps to rid your diet of GMO (genetically modified foods) and chemicals, it can become overwhelming. Pesticides and chemicals reach the food through several avenues. When you have relevant information, you can make better choices for your health.

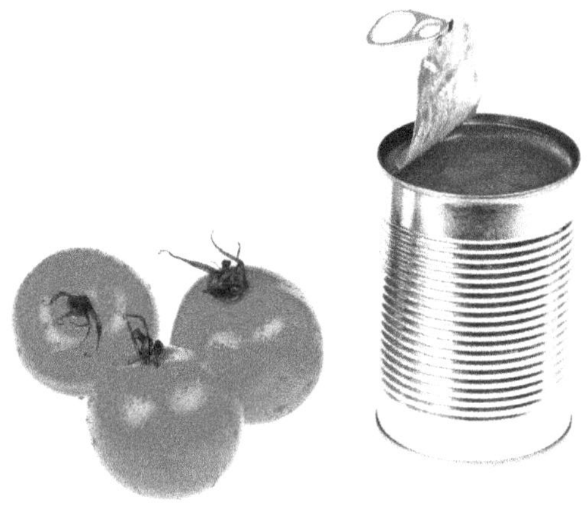

Canned Tomatoes

Tin cans' resin linings may contain Bisphenol-A, which is a synthetic estrogen linked to several ailments that range from problems of the reproductive system to heart disease, obesity, and diabetes. Acidity can cause seeping of BPA into your food. Hence, be aware of canned tomatoes. Read the labels.

Studies show that levels of BPA in the majority of the American population are actually higher than the amount known to suppress the production of sperm or that can result in chromosomal harm to eggs. Up to 50 mcg of BPA have been found in a single liter of canned tomatoes. Again, read the labels and contact the manufacturer if you have questions. Many companies are phasing out or already have eliminated BPA from their packaging.

Eat clean by selecting glass-bottled tomatoes, like Coluccio and Bionaturae brands. If possible, use pasta sauce that is bottled instead of canned. Use pasta sauces that have low sodium levels and few ingredients added.

Beef That Is Corn-Fed

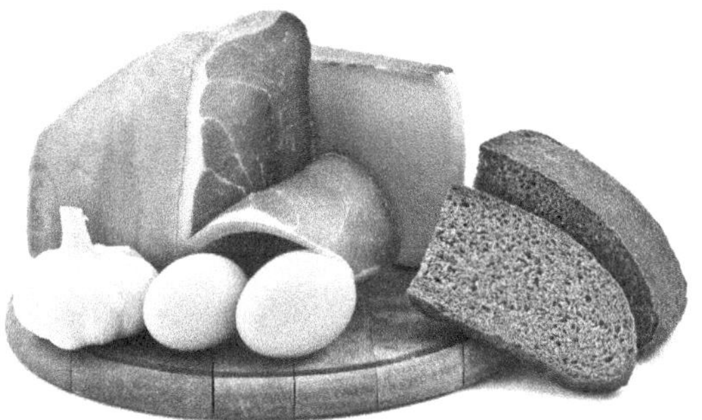

Cattle are made to consume grass, not grains. However, farmers today give their animal's soybeans and corn to eat to ensure that their animals get fat quickly so they can be slaughtered. However, the practice results in the human body getting less nutrition.

The solution is to purchase beef that has been fed with grass which is usually available at farmers' markets, specialty grocers, and at Whole Foods nationwide. It is generally labeled as grass-fed beef. If you don't see it on the label, ask the butcher.

Microwave Popcorn

PFOA (perfluorooctanoic acid) comes from a group of compounds believed to be associated with human infertility, according to a recent UCLA research. When tested on animals, these chemicals can cause cancer of the pancreas, testicles and liver. The chemicals have been shown to change to vapor in the microwave and transfer to the popcorn.

Researchers have found that these chemicals can remain in the body for several years and accumulate there. They also are concerned that the levels found in humans resemble the quantity that causes cancers in lab-tested animals. Even though some popcorn manufacturers are working to reduce and phase out PFOA by the year 2015, there will be millions of bags of popcorn consumed between now and then.

To avoid this, use the old-time method of popping natural kernels in your skillet. To add flavorings, try dried seasonings like soup mix, dill weed or vegetable flakes. Real butter can also be used.

Potatoes That Are Nonorganic

Fungicides as well as pesticides and herbicides which end up in the soil are absorbed by the roots of potatoes. Farmers treat potatoes, with fungicides in the growing season. Herbicides are then sprayed on them to get rid of fibrous vines prior to harvesting. They are further treated after being dug up to avoid sprouting.

It is best to purchase organic potatoes. Washing the chemicals from treated potatoes isn't a safety net; they are usually absorbed deeply in the flesh.

Farmed Salmon

Farmed salmon is found to have less vitamin D content and higher levels of contaminants which include PCBs, carcinogens, and pesticides like DDT and dioxin, among others. They may also be treated with high amounts of pesticides and antibiotics.

Obesity and diabetes have also been associated with DDT, but many nutritionists believe that the omega-3 content (and its benefits) far outweighs the risks

Choose wild salmon to avoid problems.

Milk That Is Produced Using Artificial Hormones

The dairy cattle of milk producers are treated with rBST or rBGH (recombinant bovine growth hormone) for boosting the production of milk. However, this component also raises the level of pus as well as udder infections in milk. It also results in higher hormone levels in milk, which have the characteristics of insulin and growth factor.

High levels of the hormone (IGF-1) have been associated with breast, colon and prostate cancers.

But according to several independent researchers, there is evidence that the casein found in milk is protective.

Even though there is no conclusive proof that IGF-1 is increasing the incidence of cancers, it is not allowed in several industrialized countries.

Ensure that you check all labels to verify that the milk you buy is free of rBGH or rBST, not produced with artificial hormones.

Conventional Apples

Apples are generally drenched in pesticides. This is because they are grafted individually in order for each variety to keep its distinctive flavor. Apples do not build up resistance to the pests that usually plague them. Therefore, they are frequently sprayed.

Although the industry holds the view that the residues will not cause harm, for clean eating, apples should be organic. If you can't afford organic, make sure they are thoroughly washed and peeled.

CHAPTER 3: CHANGING UP YOUR DIET AND EATING HABITS

Tips for Starting a Diet that is Plant-Based

Get Equipped

Find a good blender. There are plenty of affordable options. (Make sure you follow operation and care instructions to ensure the investment lasts.)

Have a good food processor in your kitchen arsenal.

Other Clean Eating Kitchen Necessities:

- A nut milk bag
- A mandolin
- A dehydrator (if your budget can manage it)

The Excalibur (9-tray) is ideal, although a cheaper model such as the Sunbeam dehydrator can be used.

Choose the Pace You Can Work With

Some people may get up one day and decide to go on a raw food only diet. But you can begin by choosing a vegetarian diet, and then steadily get rid of the foods that are known to cause harm.

Eliminate dairy slowly. It will not be easy. But there are very good soy alternatives. Be sure to monitor your calcium intake as you cut back on milk products.

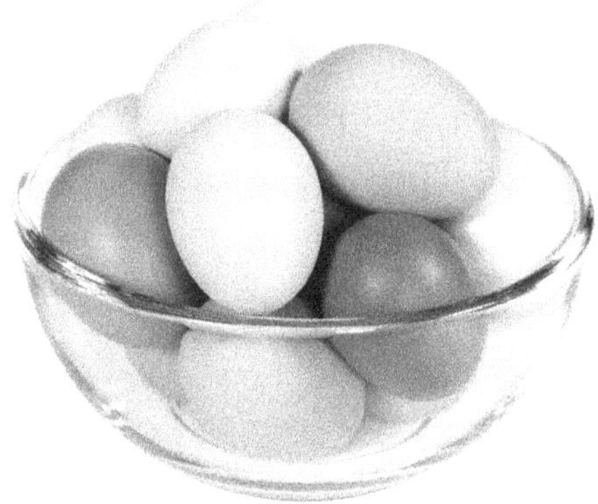

Start a Recipe Folder

When you come across recipes for raw food diets, put them in a folder. Share and compare with friends!

Look for Individuals Who Motivate You

If your main motive for trying a plant-based diet is for losing weight, look for people who you know have moved to clean eating and had positive results.

Do Not Allow Yourself to Be Deprived

Ensure that you have plenty of the foods that you love. You do not have to starve. You will not gain weight as long as you are consuming the correct foods.

What you will notice is that there will be a significant decrease in appetite as your body gets the required nutrients. Keep plenty of tasty fruits at hand for those times when you need something easy and quick. The most ideal fast food is fruit!

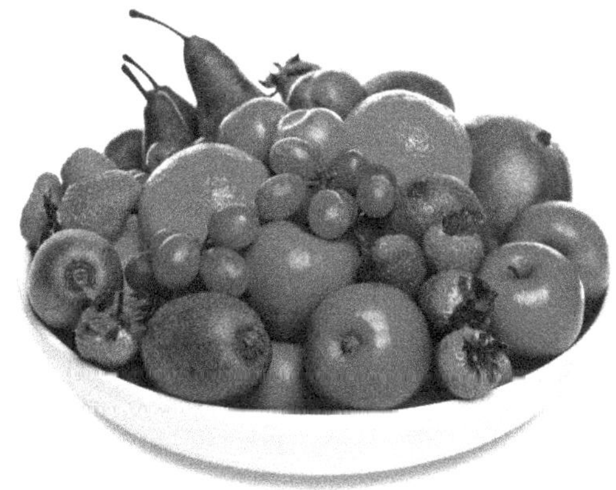

Involve Yourself in Social Networking

Do not be surprised if the majority of your family members and friends are not as excited about your change in diet as you are. You can find people on Facebook who practice (or are attempting to practice) a clean eating or raw food diet. There is ample support online.

Getting Family and Friends Involved

The simplest way to get friends and family involved is to create raw desserts. Raw desserts can be prepared without using sugar, animal products, wheat, or any other forbidden foods. You will not feel guilty making these sugary treats.

One other idea would be to invite friends for lunch and make a few enjoyable raw dishes to offer them. People usually think of boring carrot sticks and salads when they hear the words "raw food." Some tasty dishes actually include raw pasta, soups, and flax crackers with dips.

Look for Raw Food Demos or Classes

You will get the opportunity to meet other individuals in your area who share your raw food interest. Observe the preparation of new recipes, take home the spoils, along with what you've learned, and enjoy.

You can learn to make raw chocolates, crackers, green smoothies, pasta, onion bread, burgers, almond milk, chocolate mousse, museli, and more. You will see how easy and quick it is to prepare these foods, and you'll also learn their specific health benefits.

Prepare Yourself for Social Circumstances

When you're invited to social gatherings, it's advised that you carry your homemade tasty raw food with you so you can have it and also share it with others. Request an eating place that serves healthy foods when you are asked to go out to dinner.

If you are not able to choose the venue, select the healthiest option on the menu. If you slip up by eating things you shouldn't, don't punish yourself and revert to your old way of eating. Simply get back on track and continue.

Keep Track of Your Progress

When you do, it helps you remain motivated. Wear clothing that fits your figure and take some photos so that you can keep track of the difference after the weight is lost. You may also purchase a similar outfit in a smaller size for the after pictures so that you can have a good comparison.

It is also a great idea to share your progress and goals with people around you. The support will motivate you to keep going. You may also inspire others to start a clean diet when they notice your success.

Purchase Meat Only From a Butcher

There is usually a question in this case involving whether meats should be purchased from the supermarket or from the butcher.

This is because the butcher provides quality meats but the prices in the supermarkets are lower.

A butcher shop is locally owned as well as operated. The meat that butchers sell comes from many different sources and local farmers will most likely provide them with it. This meat is of absolute high quality and most of the time you can select the piece you want directly from the butcher's meat slab.

A butcher's prices are usually a bit higher. But the extra cost is worth the time and effort you save. In addition to getting quality meat, you can support local businesses.

Supermarkets are generally large chains which may have national and sometimes global reach. They get their meat from several large corporate farms. These farms may not use fair practices. The animals may be treated poorly.

Supermarket meats are generally of lower quality when compared to the meat stocked by your local butcher. Even though the prices at the supermarket are lower, the disadvantage is that you are not able to negotiate extra discounts or special savings.

The choice that is better for you will largely depend on whether you are more concerned with meat quality or with saving money.

Eating Less When You Eat More

A highly essential clean eating step starts in your kitchen. The easiest possible way to eat clean is to significantly reduce the size of your meal. It's not as difficult as it might sound. When you start eating smaller portions, your body will actually become accustomed to the change. Keep track of the amount you consume when eating a regular meal and adjust accordingly.

Analyze the amount you take in for dinner and lunch, for instance. When you finish eating, consider which portions could be reduced without minimizing your enjoyment of the meal.

A lot of times when we think we are feeling hunger, what we're experiencing is actually thirst. Before meals you can drink water, or juice that has low sugar. When it is time to eat, you will notice that you do not need as much food in order to feel full.

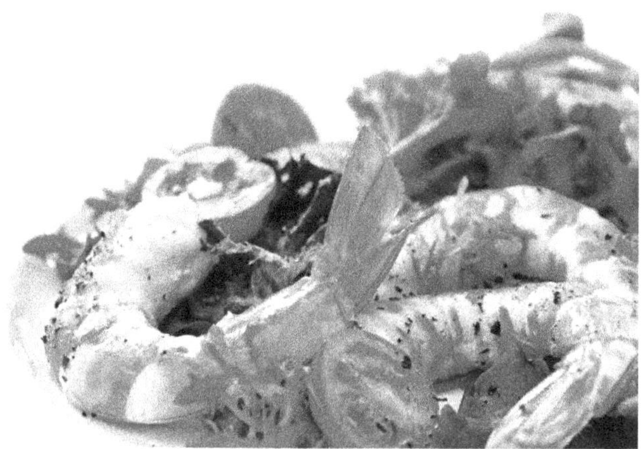

Keep note of the amount of food that is required, instead of desired, to make you adequately full. Even though you might crave some fast food, your body does not need it. One simple thing is to add more ingredients to your salads (like beans) to fill you up. You can replace several slices of pizza with a vegetable burger, or a considerable serving of whole wheat pasta, along with a salad on the side.

One or two nutritious snacks in the afternoon can help to keep the metabolism high and prevent you from feeling famished and leave you overeating at dinnertime. Snacks will help you maintain a stable energy level.

When you go out to eat, request that the waiter put a quarter or a half of the meal in a box, before you start eating. Restaurants usually serve at least twice what a person should eat. You can enjoy your saved meal portion as another meal the next day.

At home, use smaller plates. Years ago, we ate our meals on smaller plates, and we weighed less.

Clean Eating May Help Control Certain Health Conditions

If you are vulnerable to certain conditions that are diet-related (such as diabetes or high blood pressure), or your health is not in good standing, clean eating can help. And be sure to read those food labels.

If you are active and you want to maintain peak athletic performance, it is important that you track your intake of nutrients. When you achieve the required DV (daily value) of fiber, vitamins, minerals and other relevant nutrients, you're ahead of the game.

Maintain an Acceptable Weight

If your desire is to maintain, gain, or lose weight, having a clear idea of the amount of calories you need is critical. On a nutrition label, you will see the serving size suggestion at the top and the amount of calories contained in a serving. You can check the total calorie intake for a day or for a week using these basic recommendations as a guide.

Tips on Eating Foods with 10 Ingredients or Less

When possible, eat foods that have no more than 10 ingredients. It will not be easy, but it can be done. As you progress, aim for 6 ingredients or less.

Eat smaller portions of lean meat–this is much less difficult for people who are not meat lovers.

Drink lots of water or unsweetened tea only. Juice is also fine, as long as it is 100% fruit juice. Coffee can fit into a clean diet, but proceed with caution. Soda IS NOT considered clean food. By clean eating guidelines, it doesn't qualify as real food. Read the labels.

There's no argument. It may not be easy to give it up, but the weight loss and the feeling of well-being that you gain by letting it go are absolutely worth it.

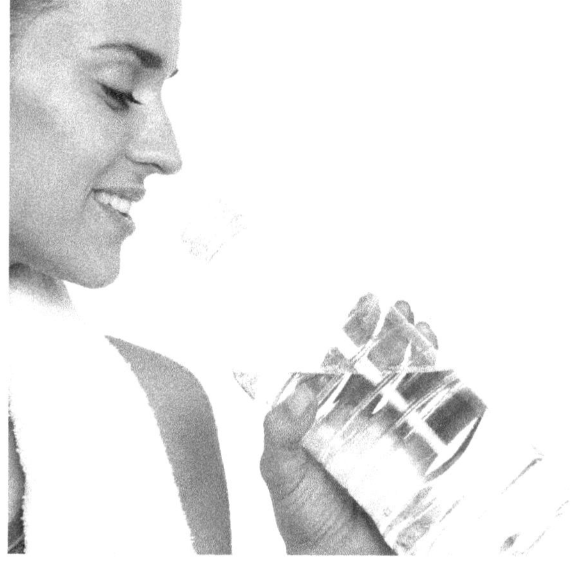

Stay very far away from fast food–if you return to it after eating clean, you'll regret that you did.

In about two weeks, you should see some weight loss and start feeling better.

Chapter 4: The Clean Eating Shopping List

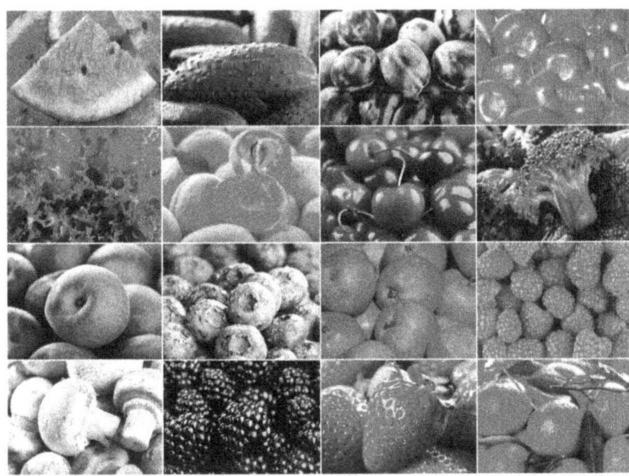

Among the number of issues people experience when they initially begin eating clean is a pantry filled with incredible amounts of junk food packed with white rice, candy, white pasta, and just about any other junk food you can imagine.

It's best to go through like a whirlwind, tossing everything in the trash and starting fresh all in one day. Switching the contents of your pantry to foods that are 100% clean may be quite a challenge. You may not have the funds to immediately start from scratch.

Each week, you can select one food that you want to replace. Candy bars can be promptly replaced with protein bars. After a few months, you'll have the perfect pantry.

APPLES

Apples do wonders for the heart and digestion. They are packed with nutrients and fiber.

APRICOTS

These little orange fruits are power-packed with health-inducing nutrients. Apricots assist in fighting cancer, slowing the process of aging, fighting Alzheimer's disease, and controlling blood pressure.

ARTICHOKES

Even though it can be difficult to eat artichokes without saturating them in mayo or butter, these remarkable green globes are known to help fight liver disease, aid digestion, and lower cholesterol.

AVOCADOS

They are incredibly delicious in a number of different dishes, and they assist in fighting high cholesterol and diabetes. Avocados can help prevent strokes. The good fats and nutrients they contain are great for your skin.

BANANAS

Bananas can assist in regulating pressure and can soothe an annoying cough.

BEANS

Beans are filled with tons of fiber. These lovable legumes assist in lowering high cholesterol, regulating unstable blood sugar, and fighting cancer.

BEETS

Either you love beets or hate them; there seems to be no feeling in between. However, if you love them, you will have a definite advantage over individuals who do not. Beets assist in controlling blood pressure, weight, and help maintain strong bones.

BLUEBERRIES

These adorable berries are a nutritional fireball. They have cancer-fighting properties. They strengthen memory and help with blood sugar and the heart.

BROCCOLI

Broccoli contains calcium, fights cancer and helps preserve good eyesight.

CABBAGE

Cabbage lovers can brag. The benefits of cabbage include heart health, cancer prevention, and weight loss.

CANTALOUPE

Assists in building the immune system and fighting high cholesterol, high blood pressure, and cancer.

CARROTS

Carrots have beta-carotene, which is great for your eyes. You will also benefit from weight loss, smoother bowel movements, reduced risk of cancer, and a better heart.

CAULIFLOWER

Cauliflower is another good source of calcium. Its nutrients defend against prostate cancer. It also fights breast cancer.

CHERRIES

Cherries preserve the health of the heart and brain and they are credited with helping insomnia and slowing the process of aging.

CHESTNUTS

Chestnuts are amazing for weight loss, lowering cholesterol, defending against cancer, and regulating blood pressure.

CHILI PEPPERS

Add heat to your meals as often as you like by adding some chili peppers to your clean eating plate. They provide better digestion, better blood circulation and a boost to your immune system. A number of studies show that chili peppers boost metabolism.

DARK CHOCOLATE

Dark chocolate is wonderful. It helps slow aging and it's great for cardiovascular health. As an added bonus, dark chocolate occupies a low position on the glycemic index.

FIGS

Figs lower cholesterol and blood pressure, and they even fight against cancer; they're a powerful ancient fruit.

FISH

Even though we need to be careful with the consumption of fish, fresh fish safeguards the heart, strengthens the immune system, and fights cancer.

FLAX SEEDS

These seeds pack a mean punch nutritionally. They assist in digestion, beef up the immune system, and help with diabetes. Chia seeds are the only thing superior to flax. However, flax seeds are far easier to access than Chia seeds and are frequently less expensive.

GARLIC

Garlic regulates high blood pressure, lowers cholesterol, kills certain bacteria, and fights cancer.

GRAPEFRUIT

Weight loss, lower cholesterol and strengthened heart have been associated with this fruit.

GRAPES

This fruit is superbly portable, so there's no reason not to include them in your diet. Grapes can strengthen eyesight as well as assist with circulation. Some studies have shown that grapes fight kidney stones and cancer.

GREEN TEA

One cup of green tea each day will help fight cancer cells and help in weight loss, as well as keep individuals from suffering a stroke.

HONEY

An old medicinal cure used for ages for various illnesses. Honey may heal wounds as well as fight allergies.

LEMONS/LIMES

Sour fruits with amazing qualities: they're known to fight the common cold and even cancer.

MANGOS

This is a tropical fruit with the ability to help with digestion and strengthen memory. Studies have shown that mangos can help in the fight against Alzheimer's disease and cancer.

OATS

Oats lower cholesterol and help in the fight against diabetes as well as improve the condition of the skin.

OLIVE OIL

It strengthens the heart, fights cancer and diabetes, and helps with weight loss. Olive oil can also be used as a skin moisturizer; all that is needed is a ball of cotton to wipe the skin.

ONIONS

Adding flavor to any dish, onions also enhance your cholesterol and makes the heart stronger.

PEACHES

Excellent for constipation and digestion.

PEANUTS

Many people are allergic to peanuts, but for those who aren't, know that consuming peanuts can help to reduce the risk of prostate cancer, heart disease, or cholesterol problems.

PINEAPPLE

Strengthens your digestive system and bones–and they help with weight loss.

PRUNES

While prunes help with memory and lowering cholesterol, they are also excellent for people with constipation troubles.

PUMPKIN

Not just for Halloween and Thanksgiving! Pumpkin controls blood pressure and it also normalizes heart function.

Rather than throwing out your pumpkins after the festivities are over, carve up the unused portion and add it to a special meal.

POMEGRANATES

These remarkable fruits have up to seven times the amount of antioxidants found in green tea and they have remarkable ability to fight cancer and reduce bad cholesterol and blood pressure.

BROWN RICE

An extremely low allergen food which protects the heart and fights against cancer and kidney stones.

SALMON

Wild salmon supplies plenty of omega-3 essential fatty acids. It is essential nutrition. Salmon also provides vitamins B12 and B3 that aid a healthy metabolism.

SPINACH

Spinach is necessary in order to grow strong. It also helps in the fight against cancer and improves brain function as well as cardiovascular health.

STRAWBERRIES

These tiny berries are easy to include in your meal plan and they are delicious! Strawberries have been shown to fight cancer and strengthen the heart. They can also be used as a natural sedative.

SWEET POTATOES

People who are clean eaters know that sweet potatoes are great carbs that can be easily included in any good clean eating plan. Sweet potatoes protect vision as well as support positive moods while keeping bones strong and healthy and helping the body fight against cancer.

TOMATOES

Known as excellent cancer fighters and they're good for high cholesterol.

WALNUTS

Great for lowering cholesterol, improving memory, and fighting cancer.

WATER

Eight glasses is known as the standard requirement each day; however this is dependent on your weight as well as your size. Water can help you to lose weight, can fight against kidney stones and cancer, and will enhance the appearance of your skin.

WATERMELON

A great summer time treat, this fruit is excellent for weight loss and it actually helps in lowering cholesterol.

WHEAT GERM

The healthiest "germ" that you will ever include in your diet. Wheat germ fights colon cancer and keeps the digestive system working smoothly.

WHEAT BRAN

Similar to wheat germ is wheat bran. It also helps defend against colon cancer and it prevents constipation. Wheat bran is also known to lower cholesterol.

YOGURT

Select non-fat Greek yogurt. Greek yogurt allows you to get more protein, in addition to reaping the benefits of increased bone strength, an enhanced immune system, lower cholesterol and better digestion. It is extremely good for ulcers.

CHAPTER 5: BREAKFAST RECIPES

They say breakfast is the most important meal of the day. Therefore it is crucially important to begin the day with a meal that is clean and nutritious, showing the hours ahead what a healthy life looks like.

GREEN CLEAN SMOOTHIE

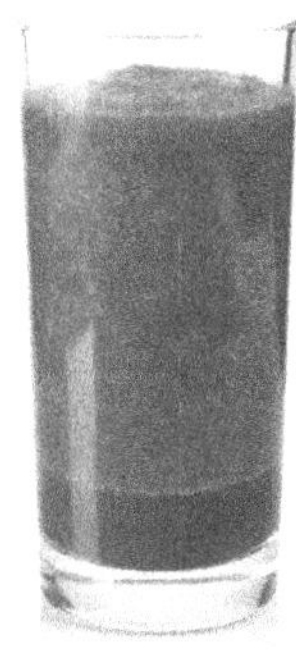

Ingredients:

2 handfuls of kale

½ cup frozen or fresh pineapple

½ banana

4 to 6 ounces. water, depending on how thick you like your smoothie

Directions:

1. Mix all ingredients into blender.
2. Blend until you have your preferred consistency.

GRANOLA CEREAL

Ingredients:

½ tsp. salt
½ tsp. ground or grated nutmeg
2 tsp. vanilla extract
½ cup honey
6 tbsp. unsalted butter
1½ tsps. ginger (ground)
2 tsps. cinnamon (ground)
1 cup raw sunflower seeds
1 cup unsweetened shredded coconut
2 cups raw sliced almonds
3½ cups rolled oats

Directions:

1. Preheat the oven to 250 degrees and use parchment paper to cover baking sheet.
2. Combine the dry ingredients in a big bowl, blending well.
3. Melt butter and honey in a pot on the stove, adding the vanilla in as well.
4. Pour the heated liquids over the dry ingredients and blend together thoroughly.
5. Spread mixture onto the baking sheet then place in the oven for 70 minutes or until golden.

AVOCADO TOAST

Ingredients:

Whole wheat bread
Avocado
Black Pepper
Olive oil

Directions:

1. Toast a piece of whole wheat bread.
2. Crush half of an avocado onto the slice and sprinkle a bit of olive oil onto it.
3. Add a dash or two of pepper

BERRY-FILLED YOGURT PARFAIT

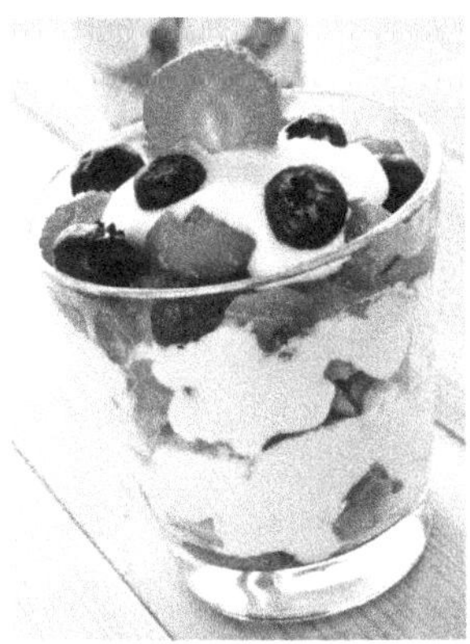

Ingredients:

½ cup strawberries

½ cup blueberries

1 cup homemade granola

1 cup plain organic yogurt

Directions:

1. Layer the fruit, yogurt and granola cereal as you wish in a glass cup.
2. Grab a spoon and run out the door with your delicious fruity treat!

WHOLE-GRAIN BANANA BLUEBERRY PANCAKES

Ingredients:

1 cup oat flour
1 cup white whole-wheat flour
2¼ tsp. baking powder
½ tsp. baking soda
¼ tsp. salt
½ cup diced walnuts
2 eggs, slightly beaten
¼ cup canola oil
1 banana, mashed
2 tbsp. honey
1 cup buttermilk
½ cup low-fat milk
½ cup fresh blueberries

Directions:

1. In a large mixing bowl, whisk dry ingredients together.
2. In another mixing bowl, combine remaining ingredients, except blueberries.
3. Pour wet mixture into dry, and stir until combined and most lumps disappear; fold in blueberries.
4. Heat griddle to 350 degrees, or until a drop of water sizzles when dropped on griddle.
5. Spray griddle with nonstick cooking spray, and pour on 1/4 cup pancake mix.
6. Turn pancakes over when they begin to dry around the edges and are golden on the bottom.
7. If desired, top pancakes with additional blueberries and bananas and drizzle with 100% pure maple syrup.

*Makes 12 pancakes

PUMPKIN MUFFINS

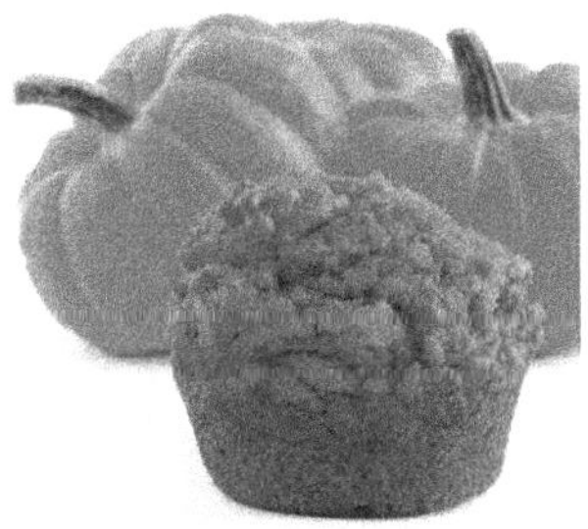

Ingredients:

1/3 cup warm water

1 cup pumpkin puree

½ cup olive oil

2 eggs

¼ tsp. ginger (ground)

¼ tsp. cloves (ground)

¼ tsp. nutmeg

½ tsp. baking powder

1 tsp. cinnamon

¾ tsp. salt

¾ cup of honey

1 tsp. baking soda

2 cups whole wheat flour

Directions:

1. Preheat oven to 375 degrees, grease a muffin pan thoroughly.
2. Combine the dry ingredients in one bowl, and the wet in another.
3. Lightly mix the wet and dry ingredients together before pouring into the muffin tins, filling each a little over 3/4 of the way full.

4. Bake for approximately 20 minutes, or until a knife used to check the middle of the muffin comes out clean.

CHAPTER 6: LUNCH RECIPES

Lunch is the perfect opportunity to take a break in your day and re-fuel your body and your mind.

ALMOND CHICKEN

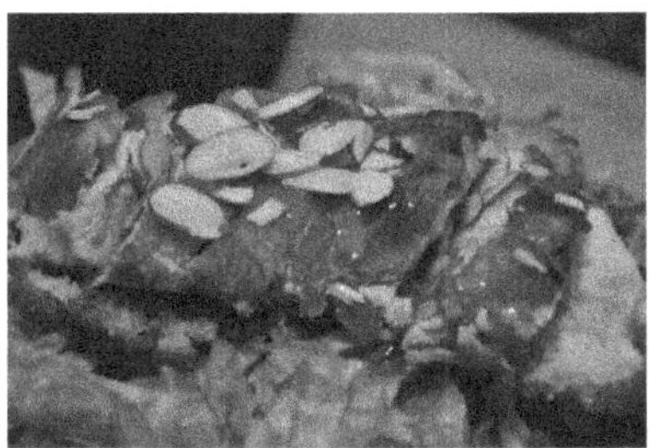

Ingredients:

4 oz. chicken breast (skinless)
¼ cup almonds
Light raspberry walnut vinaigrette

Directions:

1. Cook one 4 oz. chicken breast any way you want except for frying.
2. Once cooked, add ¼ cup of sliced almonds.
3. Add 1 tbsp. of light raspberry walnut vinaigrette.

*1 serving

CHICKEN & PINEAPPLE SALAD PITAS

Ingredients:

2½ cups chopped cooked chicken breast (about 1 pound)
½ cup matchstick-cut carrots
1/3 cup sliced almonds

1/3 cup light mayonnaise
¼ cup finely chopped green onions
¼ cup plain fat-free yogurt
1 tbsp. Worcestershire sauce
½ tsp. garlic powder
¼ tsp. salt
¼ tsp. black pepper
1 (8-ounce) can crushed pineapple in juice, drained / fresh pineapple when in season
4 (6-inch) whole wheat pitas, each cut in half / whole wheat bread
8 Romaine lettuce leaves

Directions:

1. Combine the first 11 ingredients in a large bowl and stir well.
2. Line each pita half with 1 lettuce leaf and fill each half with 1/3 cup chicken mixture.

*4 servings

TURKEY & BLACK BEAN TACOS

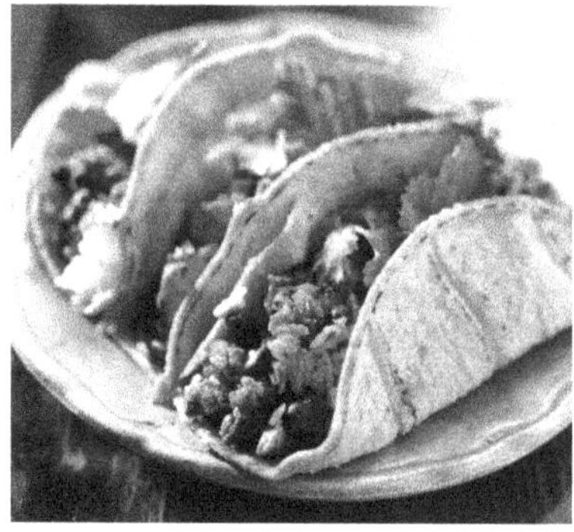

Ingredients:

Tortillas
1 pound extra-lean ground turkey
1 can low-sodium black beans, drained and rinsed
1 cup low-sodium salsa or 1 large sliced tomato

2 packed cups romaine lettuce
Sliced onion optional

Directions:

1. Coat a skillet with cooking spray. Heat the pan on medium-high.
2. Add ground turkey to the pan, and cook until turkey is cooked through, usually about eight minutes.
3. Break the meat up as it cooks, and add salt and pepper to taste.
4. Add 1/2 cup turkey, 1/4 cup beans, 1/3 cup romaine lettuce, and 2 tbsp. of salsa to a tortilla.
5. Wrap or fold the tortilla and enjoy.

ASIAN CHICKEN WRAP

Ingredients:

2 tbsp. almonds, slivers
1 6-inch whole-wheat tortilla
3 ounces skinless chicken breast
½ cup snow peas
½ cup bean sprouts
½ cup red bell pepper
1 tsp. oil & vinegar or fresh squeezed lemon juice

Directions:

1. Cook chicken
2. Cook snow peas
3. Heat a pan over medium heat. Add almonds and bean sprouts to pan. Stir until toasted (4-5 minutes).
4. Place all the ingredients into the tortilla and fold into a wrap.

*1 serving

POACHED TROUT

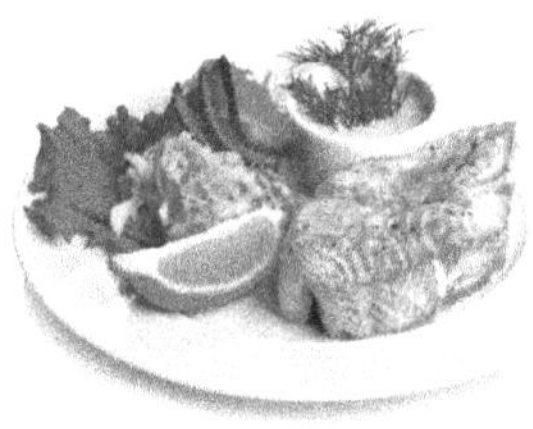

Ingredients:

1 fresh lemon, sliced
2 leeks, halved
2 cups water
1 8-ounce boneless trout fillet, skin on
Sea salt and pepper

Directions:

1. Layer lemon and leaks along the bottom of a large skillet and add water.
2. Bring to a simmer.
3. Season the trout to taste with salt and pepper and gently place it on top of the lemons and leeks.
4. Cover the skillet and simmer for eight minutes. Fish is ready to serve when it easily flakes with a fork.

CHAPTER 7: SNACK RECIPES

Small, nutritious snacks will keep your energy levels up throughout the day.

GREEN APPLE & PEANUT BUTTER

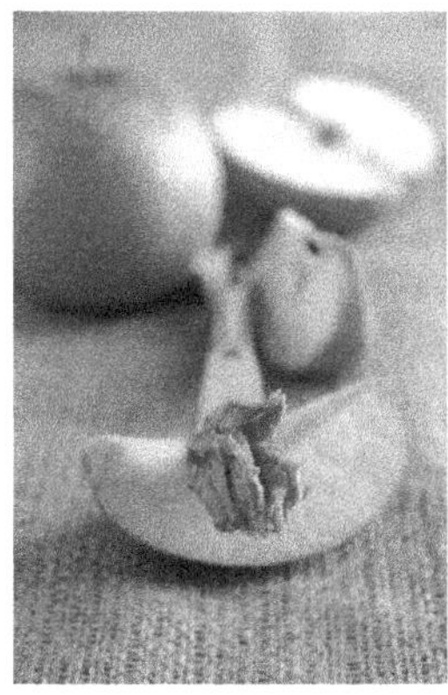

Ingredients:

1 large green apple

1 tsp. natural, creamy peanut butter

Directions:

1. Rinse apple and slice.
2. Top with peanut butter.

PARMESAN PARSLEY POPCORN

Popcorn is a favorite snack that can fit easily into the clean eating lifestyle when it is air popped and coated with flavorful, natural toppings. Here is a popcorn recipe that is sure to please any crowd.

Ingredients:

4 cups air popped popcorn

4 tbsp. freshly grated Parmesan cheese

2 tsp. minced fresh parsley

Directions:

1. Place the popcorn kernels into an air popper until popped.
2. Then, sprinkle the popcorn with the Parmesan cheese followed by the parsley.
3. This recipe can also be adjusted by adding different herbs and cheeses to suit a person's tastes.

KALE CHIPS

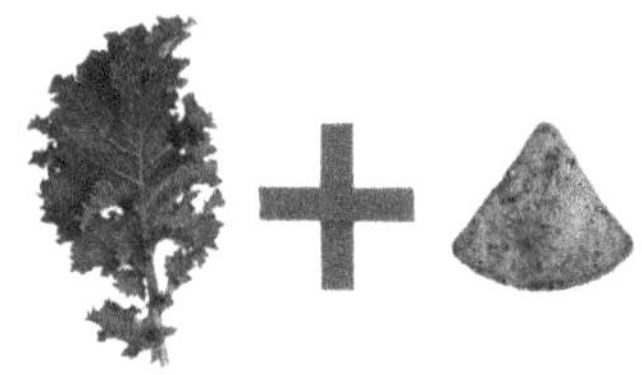

Ingredients:

1 medium bunch of kale

2 tbsp. olive oil

Pinch of sea salt

Pepper to taste

Directions:

1. Remove kale from the large stems running down the middle of the leaves.
2. Tear the leaves into two inch size pieces, and then wash them thoroughly.
3. Use a salad spinner to dry the leaves or pat them dry with a paper towel.
4. Line a baking sheet with aluminum foil and pre-heat oven to 350˚.

5. In a large bowl combine kale and olive oil. Mix with your hands until all the leaves are well coated. Add salt and pepper then toss it one more time to distribute evenly.
6. Place the kale leaves on the lined baking sheet face down so that the leaves create a small dome over the baking sheet.
7. Bake in the oven for 10 minutes. Depending on your oven, this might take slightly less or more time.
8. It is ready when the tips of your kale leaves start to turn brownish in color, and the rest of the leaves are dry.
9. Let it cool for a few minutes and enjoy.

*You can add almost any spices to your kale chips. Add cumin, red pepper, and cayenne for a spicy twist, or toasted sesame seeds, two tsps. sesame oil, garlic powder, and turmeric for a flare of Asian flavors.

OVERNIGHT OATMEAL

Ingredients:

½ cup oatmeal
1 cup non-fat Greek yogurt (plain or flavored)
Fresh fruit
¼ cup almond milk for fat-free milk

Directions:

1. Put the oatmeal in a bowl or some kind of container-I like to use mason jars.
2. Then, add the rest of the ingredients: the fruit, yogurt, and milk.
3. Mix all of the ingredients together, put the container in the fridge and cover it with plastic wrap.
4. The next day the oatmeal will be moist just as if you cooked it and the fruit will add a hint of sweetness.
5. If you use plain oatmeal, you can add some cinnamon to give the oatmeal some warmth.

TROPICAL FRUIT POPS

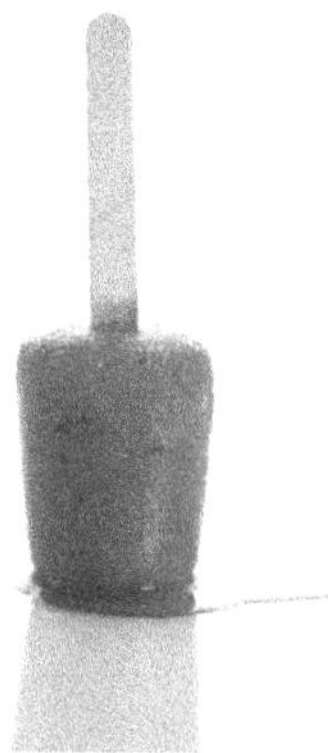

For a frozen twist on the traditional smoothie, try keeping a tray of these fruit pops in the freezer for a quick and chilly sweet treat.

Ingredients:

¼ cup pineapple
¼ cup strawberries
1 banana
1 mango

Directions:

1. Wash, chop and prep the fruit before placing it all into a blender.
2. Once processed, pour the mixture into Popsicle molds or ice trays and freeze.

Chapter 8: Salads

Salads are a great way work fiber, fruits and vegetables into your diet.

GREEN SALAD

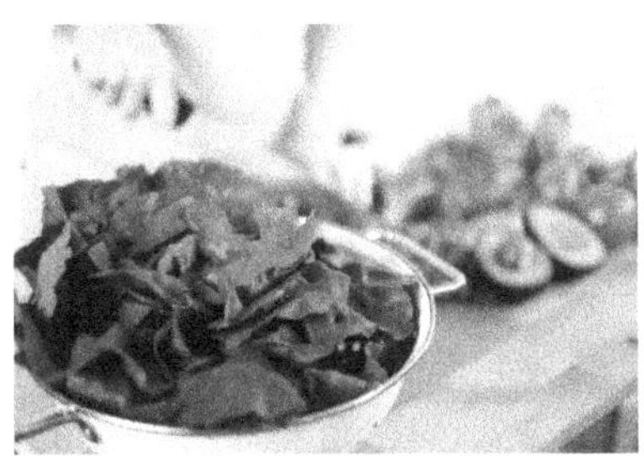

Ingredients:

1 cup lettuce of your choice
2 tsp. olive oil
1 tsp. vinegar
1 tsp. pine nuts

Directions:

1. Toss ingredients and enjoy.

CITRUS SALAD

Ingredients:

1 grapefruit
1 blood orange
2 mandarin oranges
1 ugli fruit
4 kumquats, peeled and halved
2 tbsp. fresh mint leaves, chopped

Directions:

1. Peel and separate your fruit, removing any seeds as you go.
2. Cut segments into bite-sized pieces, and place in large bowl.
3. Sprinkle fruit with mint, toss gently, and chill for 15 minutes before serving.

CUCUMBER SALAD

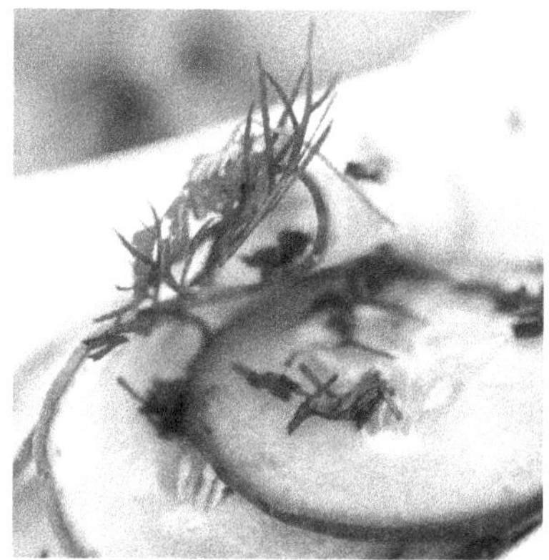

Ingredients:

4 medium cucumbers, thinly sliced
2/3 cup white vinegar
2/3 cup water
4 tbsp. sugar
1 tsp. salt
¼ tsp. pepper

Directions:

1. Thinly slice cucumbers, leaving the peel on.
2. In a separate bowl, combine the vinegar, water, sugar, salt and pepper.
3. Pour this mixture over cucumbers.
4. Cover and refrigerate for 3 hours or overnight.
5. Drain and serve cold.

CHEF SALAD

Ingredients:

2 ounces turkey

2 ounces ham

1 ounce reduced-fat Swiss cheese (optional)

2 cups mixed green lettuce

¼ cup sliced avocado

1 large tomato chopped

1 cup carrots chopped

1 tbsp. reduced-calorie ranch dressing

Directions:

1. Mix ingredients with dressing and enjoy.

HONEY BAKED SALMON SALAD

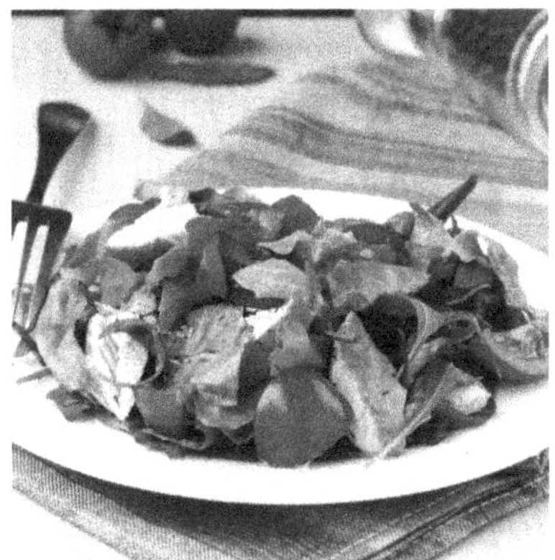

Ingredients:

4 6 ounce wild-caught salmon fillets, skinless

4 tbsp. honey

1 tbsp. extra-virgin olive oil

½ lemon, juiced

½ cup baby spinach

2 medium carrots, diced

1 medium cucumber, quartered

1 cup grape tomatoes, halved
¼ cup toasted pine nuts
Sea salt
Ground black pepper

Directions:

1. Grease a 9x13x2-inch baking pan.
2. Set oven to 400°.
3. Place salmon fillets in pan.
4. In a small mixing bowl, whisk together honey, olive oil, and lemon juice.
5. Spoon the mixture over the fillets and sprinkle with salt and pepper.
6. Bake for 10 to 12 minutes.
7. Meanwhile, prepare your salad. Divide spinach, carrots, cucumber, tomatoes, and pine nuts evenly among four salad bowls.
8. Once salmon is finished, slice into strips and place on top of each salad.
9. With a whisk, gently stir the drippings that remain in the pan. Using a spoon, drizzle a small amount on top of each salad.

PEACH AND TOMATO SALAD (Seasonal)

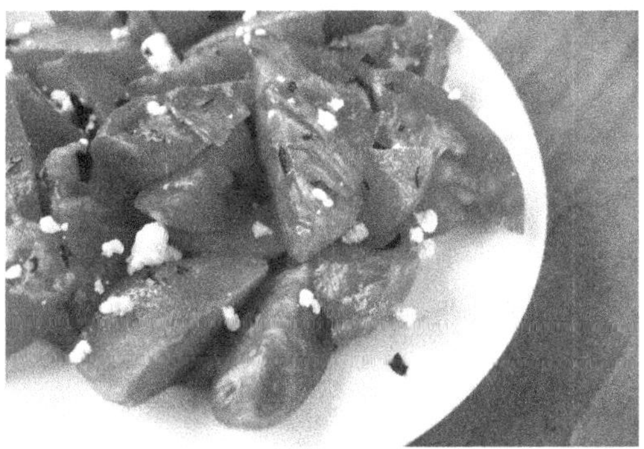

Ingredients:

¼ cup vertically and thinly sliced red onion
½ lb. ripe peaches pitted and cut into wedges
¼ lb. heirloom beefsteak tomatoes cut into thick wedges
¼ lb. heirloom cherry tomatoes halved
1 tbsp. sherry vinegar or red wine vinegar
1½ tsp. extra-virgin olive oil
1 tsp. honey
1/8 tsp. sea salt (optional)
1/8 tsp. freshly ground black pepper
¼ cup (1 ounce) crumbled feta cheese (non-fat feta optional)
2 tbsp. small basil leaves or torn basil

Directions:

1. Combine first 4 ingredients in a large bowl.
2. Combine vinegar, olive oil, honey, salt, and pepper in a small bowl, stirring with a whisk.
3. Drizzle vinegar mixture over peach mixture; toss well to coat.
4. Sprinkle with cheese and basil.
5. Refrigerate before serving.

*Pairs well with any white grilled meat

CHAPTER 9: DINNER RECIPES

Don't let a hectic and long day be an excuse for skipping a healthy and delicious meal.

PASTA AND SHRIMP

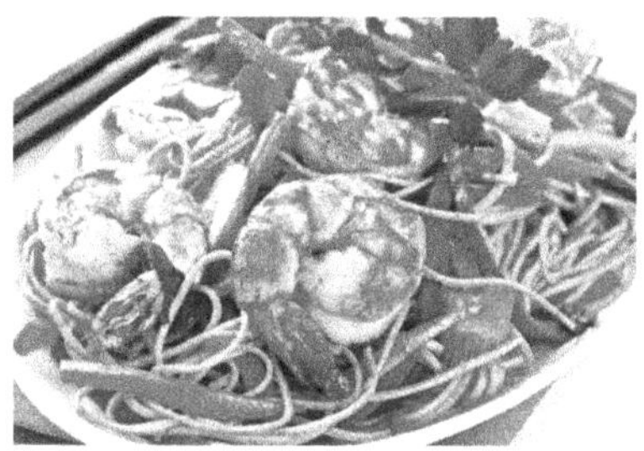

Ingredients:

2½ cups cooked whole wheat angel hair (about 5 ounces uncooked pasta)

¾ cup chopped plum tomato

½ cup chopped red bell pepper

½ cup chopped yellow bell pepper

1/3 cup chopped green onions

2 tbsp. fresh lemon juice

1 tbsp. chopped pitted kalamata olives

1 tbsp. olive oil

1½ tsp. chopped fresh or 1/2 tsp. dried thyme

½ tsp. white pepper

¼ tsp. dried oregano

¾ pound cooked medium shrimp, peeled and deveined

1 garlic clove, minced

½ cup (2 ounces) crumbled feta cheese (fat free feta optional)

1 tbsp. chopped fresh parsley

Directions:

1. Combine the first 13 ingredients in a large bowl.
2. Sprinkle with cheese and parsley.

MARINATED ROSEMARY CHICKEN AND RED POTATOES

Ingredients:

¼ cup extra virgin olive oil
3 cloves garlic, crushed
3 tsp. rosemary, finely chopped
1 lemon, juiced
8 red potatoes, rinsed and halved
4 bone-in chicken breasts, skin removed
Kosher salt
Ground black pepper

Directions:

1. Combine olive oil, garlic, rosemary, lemon juice, and a pinch of kosher salt and pepper in a resealable bag. Shake until well blended.
2. Add chicken and seal the bag. Shake once more. Refrigerate for an hour or overnight.
3. Set oven to 400°.
4. Remove chicken from the bag and place 1 breast in each corner of a casserole dish.
5. Place red potatoes in the center of the casserole dish with chicken.
6. Use a portion of the remaining marinade to lightly coat both the chicken and potatoes.
7. Bake uncovered for 35 minutes or when chicken juices run clear.

*Consider serving with a side of steamed string beans or asparagus.

SLOW COOKED BEEF STEW

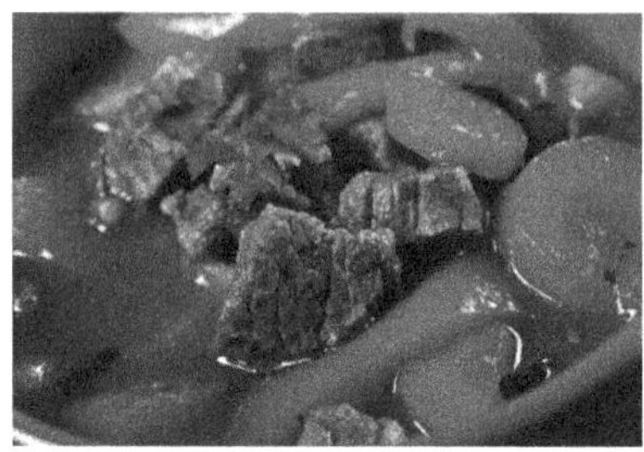

Ingredients:

1 lb. extra lean stewing beef cut into 1-inch cubes
¼ lb. low-sodium turkey bacon
1 cup onion, chopped
2 cups low-sodium beef broth
2 cups apple cider
1 lb. diced potatoes
2 medium carrots, peeled and sliced
2 ribs celery, sliced
1½ cups diced rutabaga
1 bay leaf
½ tsp. dried rosemary, crumbled
½ tsp. freshly ground black pepper
1 tbsp. freshly chopped parsley or dried parsley flakes (optional)
2 tbsp. whole wheat flour

Directions:

1. Cook beef, turkey bacon and onions in a large skillet on medium heat until the beef is browned and bacon is cooked.
2. In the slow cooker place the beef, bacon, onions, broth, apple cider, potatoes, carrots, celery, rutabaga, bay leaf, rosemary, pepper and parsley. Cover and cook 7 to 9 hours.
3. Combine flour with 2 tbsp. cold water to form a smooth mixture. Stir mixture into slow cooker and continue cooking for another 15 minutes. Serve.

*Double recipe to fit in a large cooker and have leftovers.
*Prep time is about 30 minutes.
*Cooking time is 7 to 9 hours in a slow cooker on low.

TORTILLA WRAPS

Ingredients:

3 whole wheat or low carb 6" tortillas (corn tortillas optional)
3 tbsp. hummus **recipe listed below*
1½ cups shredded lettuce
1 green bell pepper, sliced into strips
6 thin slices of avocado (about ¼ of a whole avocado)
1 large fresh red chili pepper
1 lime wedge
1/3 of a free-range chicken breast, sliced into strips

Directions:

1. Cook the chicken.
2. Rinse and shred lettuce, slice the bell pepper and chili pepper, slice the avocado, and cut the lime into a wedge.
3. Sprinkle the tortillas with water and place in the microwave on high for 10-15 seconds to soften.
4. Remove tortillas and place flat on a cutting board. Spread all three tortillas with hummus and add the remaining ingredients: shredded lettuce, green bell pepper, avocado slices, chili pepper, and sliced chicken strips.
5. Spritz with lime juice and fold in half before serving.

****Hummus Recipe***

1 can organic garbanzo beans
½ cup grape seed, coconut or olive oil
2 whole fresh garlic cloves, minced

Preparation:

1. In a small food processor, blend garbanzo beans, oil and garlic until smooth. Add a bit more oil or water if needed.

SALMON WITH LEMON & PEPPERS IN FOIL PACKETS

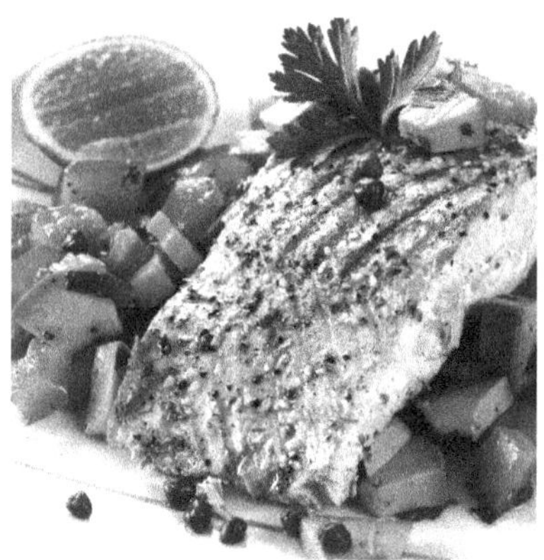

Ingredients:

2 salmon fillets

2 red or yellow bell peppers sliced

2 slices of fresh lemon

Generous amount of cracked black pepper

Pinch of sea salt

Directions:

1. Preheat oven to 370 degrees Fahrenheit.
2. Take two pieces of foil and place a salmon fillet in each one.
3. Top the fillets with the bell peppers and a lemon slice for each.
4. Add the black pepper, salt and a small amount of olive oil.
5. Seal the foil parcels and cook in the oven for 40 minutes.

CHAPTER 10: DESSERTS

At the end of the day, don't deprive your sweet tooth. Healthy and nutritious desserts can be a daily part of clean eating.

Banana Bread

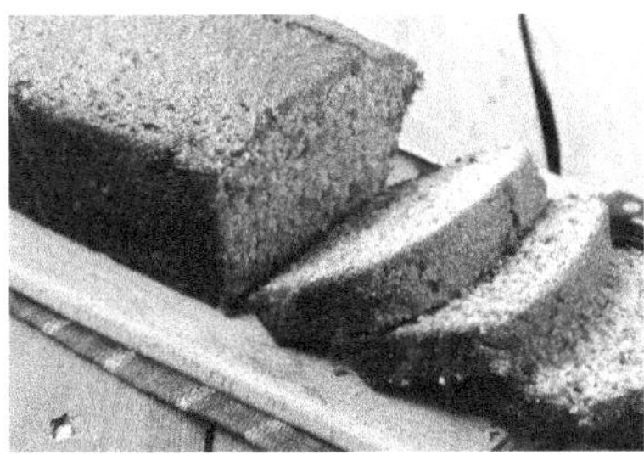

Ingredients:

1 tsp. baking soda
1 tsp. cinnamon
1 tsp. vanilla extract
1 tsp. salt
1 tbsp. soybean oil
1/3 c raw honey
1½ cup flour (whole-wheat)
3 large bananas

Directions:

1. Combine all ingredients together in a bowl.
2. Pour mixture into a bread pan and bake at 350 degrees for about 40 minutes.

CREAMSICLE SMOOTHIE

Ingredients:

3 tbsp. real maple syrup

2 tsp. vanilla extract

½ cup organic milk

1½ cups of ice cubes

1 peeled large orange

Directions:

1. Puree and blend the orange as thoroughly as possible, making sure you blend it to a smooth consistency.
2. Add remaining ingredients and blend well.
3. Pour into glasses and serve, enjoying the creamy frothiness this healthy drink creates.

LAVA CAKE

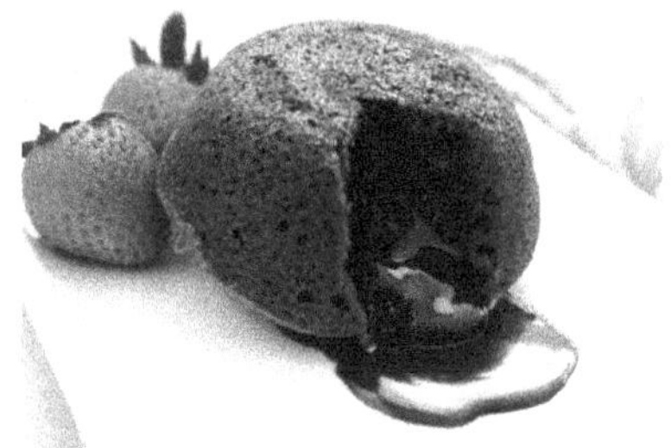

Ingredients:

Cooking spray

½ cup whole-wheat flour

1/3 cup unrefined sugar cane

¼ cup unsweetened cocoa powder

1 tbsp. vanilla extract

1 egg

1 egg white

3 tbsp. unsweetened apple sauce

3 tbsp. olive oil

Directions:

1. Preheat oven to 400 degrees Fahrenheit.
2. Coat the cake ramekins with cooking spray.
3. Combine cocoa powder and sugarcane in a bowl. Add apple sauce and olive oil.
4. In another bowl, whisk the eggs and add the first mixture to the solution.
5. Stir in the vanilla and flour until the mixture is completely smooth (don't mix too much!).
6. Pour the mixture into each of the ramekins.
7. Place each on a baking pan and heat in the oven for about 10 minutes.

CHOCOLATE CHIP COOKIES

Ingredients:

½ tsp. of salt
½ tsp. baking soda
1 cup almond butter
¾ cup unrefined sugar cane
1 egg (large)
3 ounces dark chocolate pieces

Directions:

1. Preheat oven to 350 degrees Fahrenheit.
2. Combine almond butter, sugar cane, egg, baking soda, and salt in a bowl.
3. After the mixture is blended, stir in the chocolate.
4. Place mixture in cookie-sized balls on a baking sheet.
5. Bake for around 11 minutes.

APPLES AND GINGER CRISP

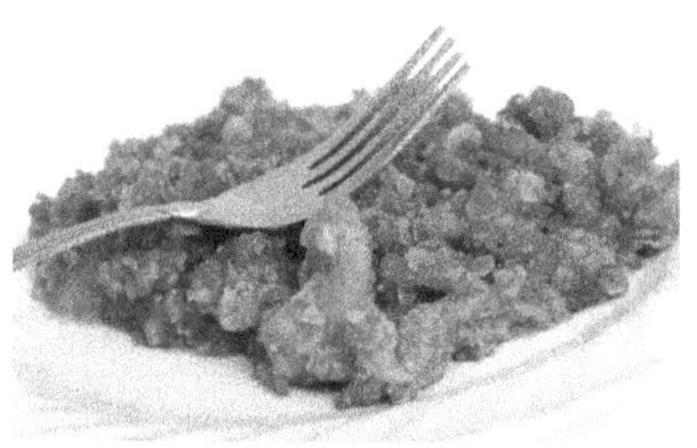

Ingredients:

1 inch ginger, minced
1/8 tsp. nutmeg
¼ tsp. cinnamon
1 tbsp. pastry flour (whole wheat)
1 tbsp. unrefined sugar cane
2 tbsp. lemon juice
6 tbsp. ground flaxseed
¼ cup water
¼ cup yogurt
1½ cup oats
1 pound thinly sliced apples

Directions:

1. Preheat oven to 400 degrees Fahrenheit.
2. Combine nutmeg, cinnamon, apples, and lemon juice.
3. Spread the covered slices evenly in a baking dish.
4. In another bowl, mix water and flaxseed and allow mixture to set.
5. Then combine flaxseed solution, ginger, and all the dry ingredients in a larger mixing bowl. Then add yogurt gradually.
6. Toss this mixture evenly over the bed of apples and bake entire concoction for about 25 minutes.

About the Author

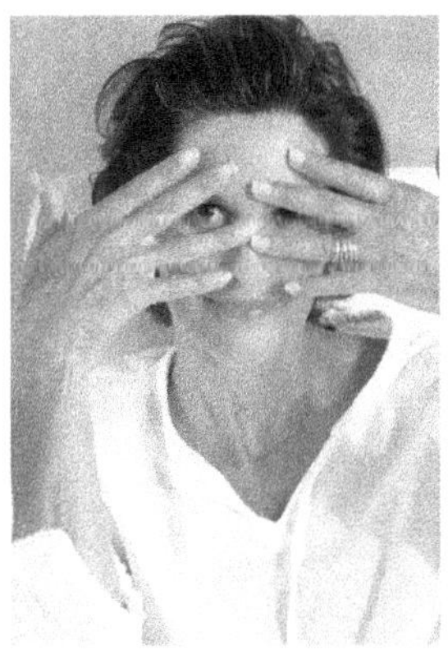

Author and chef Daisy Williams is passionate about clean and healthy eating, but she knows that it can seem next to impossible to someone just embarking on a food journey. It took years for her to move from the all-American diet processed and chemical-ridden convenience food to a healthier lifestyle that draws true nourishment from organic, whole foods. Now that she's made the transition herself, she loves helping people realize that there is a healthier way and that it's not as hard as you might think!

Eating clean didn't come easily to Daisy—her food journey started out of pure necessity. After being constantly ill for years and trying just about every medicine under the sun, she finally tried the nutrition angle as a last-ditch effort. A friend had advised reducing the chemicals in her diet, and since nothing else seemed to be working, she figured there was nothing to lose. Within weeks it became clear that nutrition was a huge factor impacting her health concerns! And thus her passion for clean eating was born.

Daisy is convinced that most people can improve their quality of life by adjusting their nutritional lifestyle. And she wants people considering clean eating to know that it's not impossible; in fact, it's delicious! Her books feature some fantastic recipes, from clean eating and green smoothie recipes that you'll love. Her dream is that through her story, people will be inspired to make healthy changes even before their health is suffering.

More Books by Daisy Williams

Clean Eating Recipes: Jumpstart Weight Loss With 70 Clean Eating Recipes -The Healthy Cookbook for the Busy Professional

Green Smoothies: The 50 Best Green Smoothie Recipes For Weight Loss – How to Make the Best Green Smoothies to Drop Pounds

Paleo Slow Cooker Recipes: The Best Paleo Diet Recipes For Your Slow Cooker

www.ingramcontent.com/pod-product-compliance
Ingram Content Group UK Ltd.
Pitfield, Milton Keynes, MK11 3LW, UK
UKHW021829270726
14058UKWH00001B/48

9 781634 280112